Meal Prep

The Ultimate Beginners Guide to Quick & Easy Weight Loss Meal Prepping Recipes - Healthy Clean Eating To Burn Fat Cookbook + 50 Simple Recipes for Rapid Weight Loss!

By *Louise Jiannes*

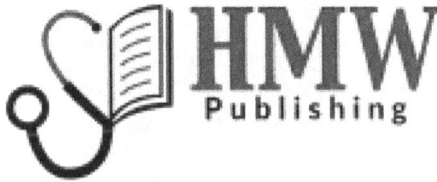

HMW Publishing

For more great books visit:

HMWPublishing.com

Get another book for Free

I want to thank you for purchasing this book and offer you another book (just as long and valuable as this book), "Health & Fitness Mistakes You Don't Know You're Making", completely free.

Visit the link below to signup and receive it:

www.hmwpublishing.com/gift

In this book, I will break down the most common health & fitness mistakes, you are probably committing right now, and I will reveal how you can easily get in the best shape of your life!

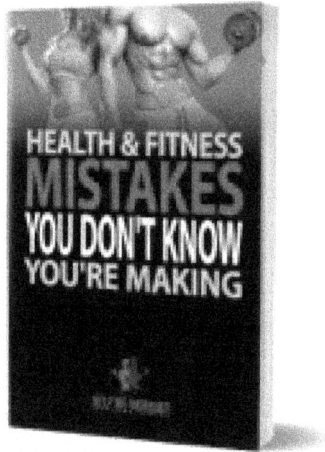

In addition to this valuable gift, you will also have an opportunity to get our new books for free, enter giveaways, and receive other valuable emails from me. Again, visit the link to sign up:

www.hmwpublishing.com/gift

Table of Contents

Introduction

I want to thank you and congratulate you for purchasing the "Meal Prep" book. Every day people are looking for solutions to eat healthily. It is never an easy task to plan meals that are not just tasty but healthy as well. However, because many are so busy in their work or taking care of their children, it becomes difficult for them to prepare healthy and nutritious meals for themselves and their family. Most of the time, they end up buying fast food meals.

Not everyone has the time and budget always to prepare mouth-watering meals in a jiffy. Others for that matter don't know how to make meals in advance because they find it hard to do. But remember, healthy eating has a lot of significant benefits that will not only be good for you but your whole family as well.

Don't fret as you are now holding the key to make healthy meals in advance! This is a great book that will help you get started in preparing nutritious meals for the whole family even if you are busy. In this book, you will learn the basics of food prepping, different foods that you can use to prep your meals in a lot of different ways and more importantly teach you to prepare them the right and nutritious way!

Meal prepping is timesaving, healthy and budget friendly. Aside from that, it is a form of habit that you can include in your daily life. There's no right or wrong way on how to prep your meals, the important thing is that you accumulate the knowledge and make use of it. The possibilities and benefits are truly worthwhile. Start reading and start prepping your meals! Have fun learning and preparing! Thanks again for purchasing this book, I hope you enjoy it!

Also, before you get started, I recommend you **joining our email newsletter** to receive updates on any upcoming new book releases or promotions. You can sign-up for free, and as a bonus, you will receive a free gift. Our *"Health & Fitness Mistakes You Don't Know You're Making"* book! This book has been written to demystify, expose the top do's and don'ts and to finally equip you with the information you need to get in the best shape of your life. Due to the overwhelming amount of mis-information and lies told by magazines and self-proclaimed "gurus", it's becoming harder and harder to get reliable information to get in shape. As opposed to having to go through dozens of biased, unreliable and un-trustworthy sources to get your health & fitness information. Everything you need to help you has been broken down in this book for you to easily follow and to immediately get results to achieve your desired fitness goals in the shortest amount of time.

Once again, to join our free email newsletter and to receive a free copy of this valuable book, please visit the link and signup now: www.hmwpublishing.com/gift

CHAPTER 1: MEAL PREP 101

When it comes to eating healthy foods, preparation is always the best key to success. One study even suggests that spending your time on cooking and preparing meals is directly linked to having better dietary habits. Meal prepping or meal prep is now becoming a popular craze worldwide. They have been going the main stream, and more people are now doing this kind of food preparation system. People who are engaged on special diets such as Weight Watchers or Paleo have been enjoying the benefits of meal prepping because it can be quite challenging to prepare their dishes especially when they are following a strict diet.

Meal prep can be different from one person to another. Hence it is essential that you will find a schedule that will work well for you and what types of food you love. But first let me show you how meal prepping has become a life changer:

- **Saves time:** the primary benefit of meal prepping is to save time. It enables you to eat healthy during the week without the hassle of preparing it for long hours. It is hard to stare endlessly in front of your refrigerator not knowing what food to make for your family. Knowing efficient meal prep can quickly help you prepare meals in a jiffy plus it will lessen the time that you need to go to supermarket just to buy your meal for the day.

- **Saves money:** some people think that to eat healthily, you have to spend a considerable amount of money. Meal prepping will prove them wrong! On the contrary, meal prepping will help save you some money because you will be able to buy bulk items and lets you utilize your freezer well. Do not be afraid to buy fresh herbs or significant amounts of chicken. There are ways to store them for future use.

- **Lets you make healthy food choices:** being busy does not give too much time for you to prepare meals at home hence the reason why most of the time you opt for fast food meals. The good thing about meal prep is that you don't have to go through eating fast food meals every day. You don't need to rely on them as a last minute alternative.

- **Shopping is made more accessible:** helps you become organized and have a list of the things that you need to prepare your meals. Making a list will help avoid buying processed foods, and sugary products that you don't need.

- **Learning portion control:** if you are following a strict diet or simply want to live a healthy life, portion control is equally necessary to be successful in your journey. Since you are already preparing for your meals in advance, you can know what food and how many calories are there in the food that you will be consuming. This will also give you a great insight into what foods are especially good for your health.

* **Adding variety in your meal:** though it may seem that meal-prepping can be quite challenging, according to statistics people who are not planning for their meal have more tendencies to eat the same food over and over again. Meal prepping, on the other hand, enables you to have a great deal of variety in your meals.

These are just some of the benefits that you can achieve once you start prepping ahead for your meals. The beauty of this is that there are no limits and no strict rules. You have the freedom to be creative and try out different meals for your whole family. The important thing is that you set aside a little time every week to do it. Once you get familiar with the system that works well with you, it would all happen in a breeze.

CHAPTER 2: GETTING STARTED

If you are new to this kind of method, here are a few of the basic things you need to know so that you can plan and get prepping for your meals.

Evaluating your eating habits

You and your families' eating habits may change every week. It will all depend on your work schedule, school activities, travel plans, commitments and another schedule that you may have lined up for the week. Consider these scenarios when making a plan:

- How many meals do you have in a day? Assess the schedule that you and your family have. Have a rough idea of each and everyone's schedule so that you know how many meals you will be preparing for the whole week.

- Time of preparing the meals: if you think that you have a busy schedule in the week to come, consider

8

looking for recipes that are easy to make or can be left out while you are working like slow cooker recipes.

- Mood: food cravings, changes in season can significantly affect your meal prep. There may be times that the food you want to prepare do not have the ingredients available because it is out of season or unavailable. Weather conditions like winter or rainy seasons need hot and warm food so try to be prepared for these kinds of a situation as well.

- Budget: think of products that are on sale and in season. Sometimes produce that is out of season can be a little expensive. So make sure that you have enough budget to carry out your meal preparations.

- A plan by writing them down with the use of a pen and paper or your apps. Jot down your planned meals, and for how many people would that be. Make sure that you also include what you can do with your leftovers.

Choosing your ingredients

Some tips that you could use in selecting some of the fresh ingredients to prepare healthy and nutritious everyday meals:

- *Look for local produce:* depending on your location, it's best to know the local food available in your market. That way, you will be able to plan the meals that you are going to prepare, and you are already familiar with ingredients that are in season in your area.

- *Meat:* Just like with fish, you would want to look for meat that is bright red. Avoid meat that already has a brownish red color. This means that it's no longer fresh. Make sure that you also smell your meat. If it smells bad, chances are, they are already there for quite a long time – don't buy it.

- *Chicken:* Fresh chicken should be pink in color. Do not buy chicken that is already grayish in color and has tears. Like meat and fish, it's essential that they don't have a funky smell. So always make sure to smell them first. For frozen chicken, check for too much blood as they can sometimes be mishandled while packaging. This increases the risk of having a lot of bacterial contamination because they could have been thawed, then frozen a couple of times.

Just a rule of thumb in choosing fresh fruits and veggies, make sure that they don't have molds, holes, brown spots or wrinkled skin. Most fresh fruits and vegetables have vibrant colors, firm and plump. You can differentiate them from the ones that are old and rotten.

Using your herbs and spices

Our food always tastes better when they are not under seasoned. However, you'll enjoy it a lot more if you know how to use herbs and spices. Be sure to season your prepped meals well to add more great flavor!

- Herbs and spices are used to enhance the flavors of our food and not to hide or disguise them. Be selective in using your herb and spice combination. Do not use too many combinations as this would only confuse or change the taste of your dish.

- For immediate release of flavor, crush herbs, like oregano, thyme, basil, in the palm of your hand before using it on your dish. This will wake up the flavors instantly.

- Dried herbs are used best when combined with oil or water because they will be infused a lot faster. Fresh herbs, on the other hand, provide full, bold flavor to your dish. This is also great for garnishing.

Compiling your recipes

Since you are already set on prepping your meals, it's now time to take a look at various recipes that you will prepare. Look for those recipes that are nutritious, healthy and your family will surely enjoy. Create a master list where you can quickly find the recipe that you will prepare. Every time that you try one, be sure to add them to your roster of recipes.

Be creative and adventurous. Look for new recipes that are worth trying and take note of them. Make sure to take note of the nutrition facts so that you will be able to meet the necessary nutrients that you need especially if you are following a specific diet. Take a look at its serving portions as well for they are essential in your meal prep. It will significantly help especially if you will be feeding your whole family. Don't forget to plan on what you will do with the leftovers.

Another good thing about meal prepping is the use of ingredients. You can select recipes that have the same ingredients which help in minimizing the amount you need to buy.

CHAPTER 3: HACKS AND IDEAS

To give you more ideas and tips on proceeding with your meal preparation, here are some excellent hacks you can try out without having to push yourself too hard!

Cook once a week

Find a day where you can take up some time to do some grocery shopping. It would be nice to do some in bulk, so you do not need to go back to the supermarket now and then just to pick something up. This might seem like a time-consuming task, but it would save you a lot of time in the future.

So take a day or even a half just to buy the things you need for cooking then chop those vegetables and meat and get ready to cook. The advantage of this is that you only need to chop once a week, preheat the oven once, and get everything ready. If it would take you around 10 minutes to cut everything you need for a meal, it would only take you about 40 to reduce those you need for 5 meals, so why not do it all today and just keep them in the freezer where they would stay fresh for at least a week.

Not only is this a time saver but electricity saving as well so you might as well consider committing yourself to cooking a batch of food once a week.

Keep it simple

No need to go and make super fancy, 5-star restaurant kind of dishes. Stay within your comfort zone and relax. Cooking is meant to be enjoyed. Do not make your life more complicated than it already is. Just keep it practical and find recipes that you would want to go and you think would enjoy making.

After all, you are trying to simplify your life by planning and preparing your meals ahead so why complicate it all by doing things that are way beyond your scope? Keep it real.

Fill that freezer

Grab those freezer bags you have or maybe some Tupperware you can write on. Store your food on your fridge to keep them from going rancid and remember to keep your fridge fool from time to time so that you do not go hungry and you are prepared for surprise guests that might come to your house.

Put that slow cooker into use

Maybe you are rushing things because you still want to go somewhere else. But keep in mind that cooking is not something to be done in a rush. It is something to be savored and loved. So why don't you put that slow cooker into use and cook some of the food you would like to see juicy, tender and delicious.

Slow cookers give you food that is just right for the taste, full of flavors and nutrition as well. Most food can even cook up to more than 8 hours so you can go to work and leave your cooker to finish cooking by itself.

Mix and match

Be creative with your food, if you seem to be missing something, just look for something else to substitute it with. Cross-utilizing your ingredients are something that an innovative chef would do so try that one out. Think about the endless combinations of food you can create by doing so.

Keep your fridge organized

You know exactly how vital your refrigerator is to you, so you must do your best to take care of it. Make some arrangement with your fridge and place it in a way that would be most convenient for you. Make it pleasing to the eyes and try to arrange it yourself so you would know exactly where anything is.

These are just some of the hacks that you can try out but do not be bound by them. Along with your journey through meal preparation, you are going to find out more hacks and maybe even create some of your own. The possibilities can be endless, and you only need to take the risk to achieve the things you want; so good luck in preparing your meals!

CHAPTER 4: RECIPES

So now that you are all set with your meal prepping, here are some great recipes that you can try out. From breakfast, snacks even mains – there is something in store for you! Get your aprons and let's get cooking!

Quick oatmeal in a jar

Ingredients

- Fruit of your choice (use freeze-dried for natural sweetness; dried blueberries; dried apples, etc.)

- Milk (coconut, cashew or unsweetened almond milk)

- Dry old-fashioned or rolled oats

Directions

1. When prepping ahead, use glass jars about a pint size. Place about ½ cup of dry oats at the bottom of the pot first. Do not use steel cut oats. Add on top your fruit combination choice then seal it tightly.

Keep in your pantry until ready to consume. This will last for around 10 days.

2. When ready to consume: pour a cup of boiling water or milk. Let it sit for around 10 to 20 minutes. Grab spoon and get ready to go!

Baked chicken and sweet potato

Ingredients

- 6 cloves of diced garlic

- 2 tbsps of olive oil

- 1 sweet potato, cut to an inch thick

- 1 ½ diced onion

- 2 cups of carrots, cut to an inch thick

- 1 lb chicken breast, cut to an inch thick

- 1 lb of steamed broccoli

- 1 tsp of rosemary, dried

- ½ cup parmesan

Directions

1. Preheat your oven to 375 degrees F.

2. Using a large baking pan, combine all the ingredients except the steamed broccoli and parmesan cheese. Season with pepper and salt then bake for around

30-40 minutes or until chicken is cooked well and veggies are also soft.

3. Remove from oven then add the broccoli and parmesan. Place on different individual containers and store until ready to consume.

Freezer Make-Ahead Sandwiches

Ingredients

- 6 pieces of large eggs

- 6 pieces of English muffins

- 6 slices of cheddar cheese

- 18 pieces of deli ham, small slices

Directions

1. Preheat your oven to about 350 degrees F.

2. Grease a large muffin tray and crack each egg on the slot. Pierce the yolk gently and add pepper and salt. Bake for around 10 to 15 minutes until cooked. Remove from slots and let cook.

3. Prepare the sandwich by layering first with cheese then about 3 slices of ham. Top with the baked egg then close the sandwich.

4. Wrap with plastic wrap then freeze until ready to consume.

5. When eating, remove from wrap then microwave for around a minute on low power. Flip then microwave for another minute.

Apple, Almond, and Cranberry Quick Salad

Ingredients

- 2 chicken breasts

- 4 stalks of chopped celery

- 2 chopped apples

- Pepper and garlic salt for seasoning

- ½ cup of almonds, sliced

- 1/3 cup of cranberries, dried

- 6 to 8 cups of mixed greens

- 2 chopped green onions

- For the dressing

- 5 oz of Greek yogurt, plain

- 1 tbsp of honey

- 1 tbsp of shallots, minced

- 2 tbsps of apple cider vinegar

- ½ tsp of poppy seeds

- Pepper and salt

Directions

1. To prepare the dressing, mix all of the ingredients and combine well. Adjust taste if necessary. Scoop around 2 to 3 tablespoons of dressing at the bottom of 4 mason jars. Set aside.

2. Meanwhile, season the chicken with pepper and garlic salt then cook using a nonstick skillet until it is cooked well. Let cool then cut to serving pieces.

3. Divide the ingredients among the mason jars. Layer in these order: celery on top of the dressing, then apples, chicken, almonds, cranberries then green onions and topmost is the lettuce.

4. Screw tightly then store inside refrigerator until ready to consumer. This will last for about 3 days.

Tofu and Zucchini Salad

Ingredients

- 2 zucchinis, spiralized

- 1 cup of carrots, diced

- 1 block of cooked tofu, cubed

- ½ cup of pitted cherries

- ½ of onion, diced

For the dressing

- 1 tbsp of tamari

- 1 ½ tsp of garlic

- 2 tbsp of rice wine

- 1 tsp of ginger

- 1 tbsp of sesame oil

- 1 tbsp of peanut butter

Directions

1. Drain any excess water from the spiralized noodles.

2. Combine carrots, onions, and cherries in a bowl. Meanwhile cooked tofu according to preference.

3. Place spiralized noodles in the bowl with combined mixture. Add the cooked tofu.

4. Using a jar, mix all dressing ingredients. Combine well. Place the veggie mixture on top then mix well once ready to consume.

Chicken with Veggies

Ingredients

- 3 pieces of chicken breasts, cut to an inch thick

- 1 chopped red onion

- 2 chopped bell peppers

- 2 chopped zucchinis

- 2 cups of broccoli florets

- 2 cloves of minced garlic

- ½ tsp of pepper

- 1 tsp of salt

- ½ tsp of red pepper flakes

- 2 tbsps of olive or avocado oil

- 1 tbsp of Italian dressing

- 2 to 3 cups of brown rice, cooked

Directions

1. Preheat your oven to 450 degrees F. line baking tray with parchment paper then set aside.

2. Put the veggies and chicken then season with all of the spices evenly. Drizzle with oil then toss lightly.

3. Bake for around 15 to20 minutes or until veggies and chicken are cooked.

4. Place about half a cup of rice in containers then divides chicken and veggie mixture evenly at the top of the rice. Cover then store in the refrigerator until ready to consume. This will last for around 5 days.

Quinoa Frittata

Ingredients

- ¼ cup of quinoa, dry

- 4 eggs

- ½ cup of water

- 1 cup of cottage cheese

- ¾ cup of diced ham

- 1 ½ cups of cheddar cheese, shredded

- 1 10 ounces pack of frozen spinach, chopped and thawed

Directions

1. Cook quinoa in boiling water covered. Reduce heat and simmer for around 10 minutes. Remove from the heat then fluff using fork then let cool.

2. Meanwhile, preheat your oven to around 350 degrees F. Spray a round pie plate with nonstick spray.

3. Add beaten eggs with the rest of the ingredients on the pie plate. Bake for around 50 minutes or until the sides become brown. Let cool for approximately 10 minutes then cut. You may also keep it in the refrigerator before consuming.

Buttermilk Pancakes

Ingredients

- A teaspoon of baking powder

- A pinch of salt

- A cup of all-purpose flour

- 1 beaten egg

- ½ teaspoon of baking soda

- A teaspoon of honey or raw sugar

- 1 ½ cups of buttermilk

- A tablespoon of melted butter

Directions

1. Combine baking powder, salt, baking soda, and flour. Mix in the egg along with the buttermilk then add it to the flour mixture. Stir well until it becomes smooth.

2. Add melted butter than sugar.

3. Using a size ¼ measuring cup, scoop the batter then fry on a griddle of about 325 to 350 degrees. This will make around 10 pancakes.

4. To store and freeze: cool it entirely after it was cooked. Line a baking sheet using a parchment paper then place the pancakes on it without touching one another. Add another layer of the parchment paper then put another pancake until all pancakes are arranged and ready to be frozen.

5. Put it in the refrigerator and freeze until it becomes stable. Once ready to use, you can heat it through toaster, microwave or grill.

Chicken Sausage with Spiralized Veggie

Ingredients

- 1 cup of crushed tomatoes, canned

- ½ tsp of Italian seasoning

- ½ tsp of powdered garlic

- ½ tsp of powdered onion

- 1 cup of sugar snap peas

- 14 oz of spiralized yellow squash

- ½ cup of onion, sliced

- 6 oz of cooked Italian chicken sausage, sliced and halved

- 1 tbsp of Parmesan cheese, grated

Directions

1. Preheat your oven to 375 degrees F then line a baking tray with aluminum foil sprayed with nonstick spray.

2. Meanwhile, combine seasonings and crushed tomatoes. Lay spiralized veggies, onion and snapped

peas on the baking tray. Top it with the chicken sausage and crushed tomato mixture. Cover with aluminum foil then seal the edges to form a packet.

3. Bake for around 20 minutes or until the veggies become tender. The open packet then transfers to containers if not eating right away.

Breakfast Quesadillas

Ingredients

- A small diced red onions

- 2 tablespoons of olive oil (divided)

- Half cup of frozen or fresh corn kernels

- ½ teaspoon of ground cumin

- ½ teaspoon of salt (divided)

- A clove of minced garlic

- ¼ teaspoon of paprika (smoked)

- 8 large-sized eggs

- A pinch of black pepper

- A tablespoon of milk

- 10 pieces of large flour tortillas

- 1 (15 oz) canned black beans (rinsed and drained)

- ½ cup of salsa (chunky style; add 2 tablespoons more)

- 1 ½ cup of shredded cheese (depends on your preference)

- Greek yogurt, sliced avocado, chunky salsa (this is optional)

Directions

1. In a large-sized skillet, add a tablespoon of olive oil over medium heat. Add onions and cook while stirring them occasionally for about 2 minutes. Add the corn, cumin, ¼ teaspoon of salt, garlic and paprika. Cook for about 3-4 minutes then transfer to a bowl. Set it aside.

2. Whisk together the milk, eggs and remaining pepper and salt. Place the skillet again over low to medium flame. Add the remaining tablespoon of olive oil. Once hot, add egg mixture and cook for around 3 to 4 minutes while stirring occasionally until it becomes scrambled. Remove from the heat.

3. Drain excess water from the bowl of veggie mixture if there are any. Add them to the skillet with the eggs. Add the black beans the combine well. Season to taste.

4. In your working station, place a tortilla and spoon about 1/10 of egg mixture on the half side of the tortilla, make sure that you leave a small space to allow folding.

5. Top it with cheese, and a tablespoon of salsa then fold the empty half on top of the filling. This should look like a semi-circle. Repeat the same process on the remaining tortilla.

6. To cook, add a small amount of oil or cooking spray on a non-stick pan. Place the prepared tortilla and cook around 5 to 6 minutes until both of the sides are browned and cheese melted. Repeat until all tortillas are cooked.

7. Cut into triangles then serve hot. This will make 10 quesadillas.

8. For make-ahead meals: cook the eggs and veggies as directed then let cool. Assemble them the same way but instead of cooking, wrap each of the quesadilla using a plastic wrap. To prevent it from bending, place them in a container with a flat surface. Put in the freezer until it becomes firm. Once firm, transfer in an airtight container, then store it back in the freezer.

9. Once they are ready to be eaten, remove the plastic wrap, warm it in a microwave for about 2-3 minutes until it is thoroughly heated. Another way of heating it is to thaw them first then cook in the skillet as mentioned in the recipe.

Berry-Berry Blue Breakfast Bars

Ingredients

- 1 ½ cup of 100% pure rolled oats

- ¾ cups of almonds (whole)

- ½ cup of blueberries (dried)

- ½ cup of pistachios

- 1/3 cup of flaxseed (ground)

- 1/3 of walnuts

- 1/3 cup of pepitas

- ¼ cup of sunflower seeds

- 1/3 cup of pure honey (you can also use maple syrup)

- ¼ cup of apple sauce (unsweetened)

- 1 cup of almond butter

Directions

1. Place wax or parchment paper in an 8x8 baking pan leaving the paper hang over the edges.

2. Combine rolled oats, almonds, blueberries, pistachios, flaxseed, walnuts, pepitas and sunflower seeds in a large sized bowl and mixed them all.

3. Slowly add the honey and continue to stir lightly. Then add the almond butter and mix them well.

4. Place the batter mix in the lined baking pan and press it firmly using the palm of your hands or if you have a mini roller, you can use that as well. Make sure that it's evenly distributed and rolled.

5. Freeze for about an hour. Remove from the freezer and slowly lift the paper with the portion of the mixture. Gently peel the paper and slice it diagonally to long bars, this would make at least 8 bars. Cut them in half to create 16 bars. Place them in a resealable bag and put them in the freezer.

6. When you are in a hurry, just get a piece and voila! Makes 16 delicious bars.

Chicken and Garlic Lime Kebabs

Ingredients

* ¼ cup of EVOO (extra virgin olive oil)

* 2 cloves of minced garlic

* A teaspoon of pepper

* A teaspoon of salt

* 4 chicken breasts (boneless and skinless cut to 1 ½ inch)

* 1 piece of lime (juiced)

* 1-2 teaspoons of Sriracha (if desired)

* Skewers

Directions

1. Combine lime juice, EVOO, pepper, salt, garlic, and Sriracha. Pour over chicken and place it in a Ziploc or resealable bag. Marinate for about 2-8 hours inside the refrigerator.

2. Remove the chicken and thread it on the skewers.

3. Preheat your grill to medium to high heat.

4. Cook chicken for about 10 to 15 minutes. Turn in once in awhile until chicken is cooked thoroughly.

5. To store, place the raw chicken in the freezer. Make sure that your resealable bag is freezer safe. Once ready to cook, thaw first. Servs of 4.

Veggie Taco Salad

Ingredients

For the cilantro and lime dressing

- Juice from a lime

- ½ cup of loosely packed fresh cilantro

- A tablespoon of apple cider vinegar

- A teaspoon of honey

- A pinch of salt

- ¼ cup of Greek yogurt (non-fat and plain)

For the salad

- ½ cup of black beans

- ¼ diced cucumber

- ¼ cup of corn

- 3 cups of mixed greens

- 1 piece of diced roma tomato

- ¼ cup of diced red pepper

- A tablespoon of cheddar cheese (shredded)

- ¼ of diced avocado

Directions

1. Prepare the salad dressing by blending the ingredients all together. Pour it into the bottom of your mason jar, about a quart size. Use those wide-mouth jars)

2. Layer the ingredients in this order: cucumber, black beans then tomato, corn then the red pepper, mixed greens, avocado and the cheese.

3. Cap it tightly with the lid and place on the refrigerator. This can be stored for 5 days. You can also choose to crush a few tortilla chips on top when you eat it.

Baked Fish Sticks

Ingredients

- 1/3 cup of EVOO

- 3 pieces of large eggs

- 3 cups of Panko bread crumbs

- A tablespoon of seafood seasoning

- 2 ½ lbs of tilapia fillets (skinless and cut to inch strips)

- Kosher salt

- Ketchup and coleslaw to serve

Directions

1. Preheat your oven to 450 degrees F. Using a large-sized rimmed baking pan, place the bread crumbs along with the seafood seasoning, half a teaspoon of salt and oil. Toast inside the oven, tossing it once, for about 5-7 minutes or until it becomes golden brown. Transfer to a bowl.

2. Meanwhile, beat eggs with a tablespoon of water. Dip the fish on the eggs and coat it with the toasted bread crumbs. Shake excess crumbs then place it on a baking pan lined with parchment paper.

3. Bake for about 12-15 minutes or until opaque and crispy. Serve it with ketchup or coleslaw if you like.

4. Uncooked fish sticks can be frozen and stored for 3 months. Freeze them first on a baking sheet until it becomes firm. Transfer to freezer bags and keep in refrigerator. Once you are ready to cook, bake frozen for about 18-20 minutes. Serves 8.

Veggie and Grilled Chicken Bowls

Ingredients

- 16 oz of cooked quinoa

- 4 cups of chopped roasted asparagus

- 4 cups of cauliflower (roasted)

- 4 cups of broccoli florets (roasted)

- 16 oz of cooked brown rice

You can also replace the veggies with:

- 4 cups of Brussels sprouts (roasted)

- 4 cups of haricot verts

For the grilled chicken

- A teaspoon of kosher salt

- A teaspoon of ground cumin

- ½ teaspoon of garlic salt

- ½ teaspoon of smoked paprika

- ½ teaspoon of ground pepper

- 2 pieces of lime

- 3-4 pieces of medium sized chicken breasts (boneless)

Directions

1. To prepare the chicken: Preheat your grill. Combine pepper, salt, paprika, cumin and the garlic salt in a bowl. Pour them over the chicken and place it in a Ziploc or resealable bag. Squeeze the juice of lime inside and marinade for about 1 to 5 hours. You can also grill it immediately. Spray some cooking spray on the grill and cook chicken for about 5 to 6 minutes on each side or until chicken is cooked thoroughly. Let rest for about 10 minutes. Slice chicken thinly and squeeze some more lime juice on top of the chicken.

2. To prepare your veggie bowls, get containers that have the same size. Place ¼ cup of quinoa and rice on each of the containers. Top it with 1 ½ cups of roasted veggies then add in about ½ cup of sliced chicken. Store in the refrigerator and reheat when ready to eat. You can add a low-fat dressing, salsa or hot sauce of choice once heated. Serves 8.

3. In roasting your veggies, place on a large sized baking sheet then drizzle it with EVOO and season to taste with pepper and salt. Cook in your oven over a 375 degrees F until it becomes tender.

Orange Chicken

Ingredients

- Juice of 3 oranges

- 3 tablespoons of fat, preferably coconut oil

- 1 teaspoon of fresh ginger

- Zest from 1 orange

- 1 teaspoon of chili garlic sauce

- 3 tablespoon of coconut aminos, Note: you can substitute with wheat-free soy sauce

- 1 pound of chicken breast, already cut into bite-size pieces

Directions

1. Combine the zest, orange juice, coconut aminos, ginger, and chili garlic sauce in medium size sauce pot over medium heat. Let it simmer for a while.

2. While letting the first ingredients to simmer, heat 3 tablespoons of fat in a sauté pan over medium-high

heat. Add all the chicken breast and let it cook until the color becomes brown and a crust has already formed in each chicken piece.

3. You can now add the chicken to the sauce pot you have prepared a while ago and stir for it to absorb the orange goodness of the orange sauce. You can also let it cool down for a while (at least for 30 minutes) and then preserve it in the freezer. Just reheat in the oven if you are now ready to eat. Serves 4-6.

4. Note: if you are not satisfied with the orange taste, try adding more zest until the desired flavor is attained.

Burrito Bowl

Ingredients

For quinoa:

- 2 cups of water

- ½ teaspoon of salt

- 1/4cup of fresh cilantro (chopped)

- Zest and juice of a lime

- A cup of quinoa

For chicken

- 2 teaspoons of sea salt

- 2 pieces of large-sized chicken

- A tablespoon of ghee or coconut oil

Other ingredients

- 2 pieces of bacon (if desired)

- A large sized sweet potato (washed and cut to half an inch cube)

- A tablespoon of bacon fat (you can also use coconut oil)

- ¾ cup of shredded cheese

- 5 tablespoons of Greek yogurt (plain)

- 3 cups of chopped lettuce

- ½ cup of fresh cilantro

Directions

1. To prepare the quinoa: add water, salt, and quinoa in a pot and bring to boil. Cook and cover for about 20 to 25 minutes or until it becomes fluffy and soft. Let cool and set aside. Once cooled, add lime juice and zest then the ¼ cup of cilantro. Stir to combine well. Add additional lime and adjust taste according to liking.

2. To prepare the chicken: pat dries the chicken breast and season each side with salt. Using a large-sized

pan heat over medium to high heat. Cook chicken around 4 minutes on each of its side or until it becomes brown. Let cool and cut chicken into small chunks. Set aside.

3. Cook the bacon until crispy. Reserve the oil and use it to cook the sweet potatoes. Sear and stir every 3 to 5 minutes. Turn heat to low and continue cooking sweet potatoes until it becomes fork tender. Cool and set aside.

4. To assemble your burrito bowl: once all of the ingredients are cooled, add a tablespoon of Greek yogurt at the bottom of the jar. Top it with around 2 tablespoons of cooked sweet potatoes. Then top it with 3 to 4 tablespoons of the quinoa mixture and layer it with cheese, then a little of crumbled bacon then chicken. Fill it up with salad greens and top it with chopped cilantro before closing lid. Can make at least 5 salad jars.

Freezer-Friendly meatballs

Ingredients

- 1 sprig fresh rosemary, minced

- 2 garlic cloves, minced

- 1 long sprig fresh oregano, minced

- 3 sprigs fresh thyme, minced

- ½ small yellow onion, already chopped

- ¼ cup flat leaf parsley, already chopped

- 2 medium-sized eggs, already whisked

- ½ cup of almond meal

- Black pepper

- 1 teaspoon of red pepper flakes

- ½ cup of parmesan, already finely shredded

- ¼ cup of cream, Note: this is optional.

- ¼ cup of bacon fat

- 1 pound of ground beef

Directions

1. In a medium-sized bowl mix all the ingredients (except the bacon fat) until they are all combined. Using your bare hands, roll and make meatballs. Tip: you can freely turn them into your desired sized but is much better to make them medium in size to cook better.

2. Over medium to medium-high heat, heat the bacon fat in a sauté pan and wait until it's hot enough. You can now add the meatballs and let them fry for about 7 minutes or wait until the bottom is already brown.

3. After cooking on one side, turn the meatballs on the opposite side for the other hand to cook. Wait until that side is also browned. This will take for about another 7 minutes. Put the meatballs on a plate after being cooked. Serve and enjoy! And of course, let the others cool down first and freeze them for you eat them on any other day.

4. You can cut one meatball in the center and see if it's fully cooked on the inside. If not, just turn the heat to low and let it stay for a few more minutes. It's also inevitable that you'll be able to make many meatball pieces and you can't cook them all at once. The trick is to cook them in batches, and the put the prepared quantities in a warm oven (to keep it hot) while the other batch is fried. This recipe makes about 30 meatballs.

Fennel and Sausage Ragu

Ingredients

- 6 cloves of garlic (minced)

- 2 small white onions (diced)

- 2 small fennel bulbs (diced)

- 2 (32 oz) diced tomatoes, include its juices

- 1 (15 oz) canned tomato puree

- A pound of hot Italian sausage

- EVOO

- 1 sprig of rosemary

- Pepper and salt to taste

- Cooked pasta (for serving)

- Grated parmesan cheese (for serving)

Directions

1. Crumble and sauté sausage with olive oil using a deep pan or Dutch oven. Brown sausage for around 10-15 minutes and continue to stir and scrape. Don't worry if it sticks at the bottom of the pan. It will be used as you cook along the way.

2. Add the diced onions, fennel, and minced garlic. Stir well to combine the sausage with the veggies. Turn the heat down and cook veggies with sausage for about 15 minutes. Once the veggies are tender, add canned tomatoes and tomato puree. Stir and simmer on low to medium heat. Add salt, black pepper, and the rosemary sprig. Continue simmering and loosely cover the pan. Take off the lid after an hour and adjust taste according to your liking.

3. Ladle a good amount of ragu over your cooked pasta and sprinkle it with cheese and fennel fronds on top. You can refrigerate this ragu for about 5 days and keep frozen for a few months. Makes about 8 servings

Stir-Fry Frozen Dinners

Ingredients

For the base to be stir-fried:

- A pound of chicken thigh or breast (you can also use other proteins such as tofu, beef or pork)

- ½ cup of uncooked brown or white rice

- 2 cloves of smashed garlic

- 1 bell pepper (chopped)

- A cup of sugar snap peas (you can also use other veggies)

For the sauce

- 2 tablespoons of dry sherry

- 2 tablespoons of soy sauce

- 2 tablespoons of water (you can also use vegetable or chicken broth)

- A tablespoon of vinegar (rice wine)

- A teaspoon of sesame oil

- A teaspoon of cornstarch (if you want to have thicker sauce)

Directions

1. Prepare rice according to the instructions on the package. Once done, spread rice over a baking pan and let cool. Transfer using a container or freezer bag. Refrigerate and set aside.

2. Add chicken, bay leaf, and garlic to a pit. Add water, making sure that chicken is covered with few inches of water. Poach and cook chicken on medium to high heat. Let it boil. Once boiling, lower the heat then cover the pot and continue to cook for about 10-13 minutes or until chicken is cooked through. If you are using tofu, it does not need to be pre-cooked.

3. Once the chicken is cooked, cut into uniform slices and transfer on a baking sheet lined with parchment paper. Make sure to leave room for the veggies.

4. Cut the veggies with the same size as the chicken then place them beside the chicken. Freeze chicken and vegetables until it becomes solid for about 4 hours. You can also do it overnight. Once frozen solid, pack them into freezer bags and make sure to press out air as much as possible.

5. Prepare the sauce by whisking together all of the ingredients. Pour them into a freezer bag and be sure that bags don't have leaks or holes. Again, make sure to press out air as much as possible.

6. Pack all the ingredients together: the rice, sauce, chicken, and veggies, in a large sized freezer bag or container. Label them accordingly and seal it without too much air as possible. They can be stored for 3 months. This serves 2.

7. To heat your stir-fry meal: defrost the sauce first. Transfer rice to a microwaveable container which is covered loosely and heat for around 2 minutes. You can also incorporate the rice while cooking the chicken and veggies in work.

8. Meanwhile, add 2 teaspoons of oil in a large-sized pan. Add chicken and cook for about 4-6 minutes. Add veggies and cook. Stir occasionally until it is warmed through and crisp-tender. Mix the sauce and stir-fry until sauce thickens. Serve on top of the rice.

Mini Parfaits

Ingredients

- 5 teaspoons of honey (clover)

- 1 ¼ cups of Greek yogurt (vanilla)

- 1 ¼ cups of frozen berries

- 5 tablespoons or more of your preferred granola mix

- Mason jars

Directions

1. Divide all the ingredients equally on 5 (4 oz) mason jars. Place the fruit first on the bottom then honey, the granola mix and finish it up with yogurt. Cover with the lid and store in the refrigerator. This can last for around 3-5 days.

Healthy Snack Bin

Ingredients

- Baby carrots

- Red grapes

- Strawberries

- String cheese

- Apples

- Trail mix of your choice

Directions

1. Place all the ingredients in different packages. To keep the berries fresh, rinse them in water and vinegar mixture, 1 part vinegar (either apple cider or white) and ten parts of water. Then place in a freezer package. Store in the refrigerator until ready to consume. The amount of these snack bins will depend on how much you want to prepare and how long you want it to last.

Sesame Crusted Chicken Bowls

Ingredients

- 12 ounces of asparagus, trimmed

- 1 cup of sesame seeds

- ½ tsp of powdered garlic

- 2 cups of cooked quinoa

- 3 bells peppers, cut to strips

- 1 lb of chicken tenders

- 3 tbsps of olive oil

- Pepper and salt for tasting

- Sesame seeds

- Red pepper flakes, optional

Directions

1. Heat a teaspoon of oil then cooks bell pepper for around 3 to 4 minutes. Set aside.

2. Cook the asparagus in the same pan the season with pepper, powdered garlic, and salt. Cook for around 5 minutes or until tender and bright green. Set aside.

3. Meanwhile, season chicken tenders with pepper, salt, powdered garlic, and oil. Coat firmly with the sesame seeds.

4. Using the same pan once again, add more oil if needed then cook chicken tenders for around 4 to 5 minutes on each of the sides.

5. Assemble the food in separate containers by dividing the quinoa then add chicken, asparagus, and bell pepper alongside. Store in the refrigerator for about four days.

Chicken Chipotle Chili

Ingredients

- 4 cloves of minced garlic

- 2 lbs of chicken breasts (boneless and skinless)

- 2 tbsps of olive oil

- 1 (12 oz) beer

- 1 can of (14 oz) diced tomatoes

- 1 can of (14 oz) black beans

- 1 can of (14 oz) kidney beans

- 1 tbsp of cumin, ground

- 3 pcs of minced chipotle peppers (adobo sauce)

- 1 tbsp of powdered chili

- ¼ cup of Masa Harina

- 1 juice of a lime

- Cilantro and lime wedges for serving

- Cheddar cheese, grated

- Sour cream

Directions

1. Heat olive and sauté garlic and the onions. Cook until soft. Add in chicken then cook until browned lightly. Add three-fourths of the beer and reserve the other. Cook for a bit more than reducing.

2. Add chipotle, powdered chili, tomatoes, salt and cumin. Stir in to combine. Cover and cook for about an hour.

3. Meanwhile, mix the masa harina with the rest of beer then stir until it makes a paste. Add the chili then lime juice. Cook for an additional 10 minutes or until the sauce becomes thick. Serve with the cilantro, cheese, sour cream and lime.

Baked Zucchini Snack Chips

Ingredients

- 1 piece of large zucchini

- Kosher salt

- 2 tbsp of salt

Directions

1. Preheat your oven to 225 degrees F.

2. Line 2 baking trays.

3. Slice zucchini with about 1-2 inch in thickness. Place on paper towels and try to squeeze excess liquid to help cook the zucchini a little faster.

4. Place on the baking tray. Do not crowd. Brush each chip with oil then season with a bit of salt. Avoid over seasoning because it might taste salty.

5. Bake for around 2 or more hours or until they are crisp and not soggy. Let cool. Then keep in airtight containers for approximately 3 days only.

Peach Melba Ref Oatmeal

Ingredients

- 1/3 cup of skim milk

- 1 tsp of chia seeds, dried

- ¼ cup of rolled oats, uncooked

- ¼ cup of Greek yogurt, non-fat

- 2 tbsps of raspberry jam

- ¼ tsp of vanilla extract

- ¼ cup of chopped peaches

Directions

1. Using a mason jar, add milk, yogurt, oats, vanilla extract, jam and chia seeds. Cover with the lid and shake well until thoroughly combined. Remove the top then add peaches. Still well.

2. Cover once again then refrigerate overnight or until ready to consume. Serve chilled. This will last for 3 days.

Breakfast Quinoa Bars

Ingredients

- 1 ½ cups of cooked quinoa

- ½ cups of chopped nuts

- 1 cup of whole wheat flour

- 1 tsp of cinnamon

- 2 tbsps of chia seeds

- 1 tsp of baking soda

- 2/3 cups of peanut butter

- 2 eggs

- ½ cup of honey

- 1 tsp of vanilla

- 1/3 cup of chocolate chips (optional)

- 1/3 cup of raisins

- 2/3 cup of applesauce

Directions

1. Combine the quinoa, vanilla, applesauce, peanut butter, eggs, and honey in a bowl. Mix well. Add the remaining ingredients then stir until mixed well.

2. Spoon the mixture on a greased baking tray then bakes for around 20 minutes on a 375 degrees F.

3. Let it cool then cut to bar size. Store in the refrigerator until ready to eat.

Bacon Choco Chip Cookies

Ingredients

- 2 cups of almond flour
- ¼ teaspoon of salt
- ¼ teaspoon of baking soda
- 6 tablespoons of melted coconut oil
- 4 tablespoons of honey
- 2 teaspoon of vanilla extract
- 2 tablespoons of coconut milk
- 4-6 tablespoons of bacon (crumbled and cooked)
- ½ cup of chocolate chips

Directions

1. Preheat your oven to 350 degrees.
2. Meanwhile using a parchment paper, line the cookie tray.
3. Combine almond flour, salt, and baking soda. Mix them well using a fork.

4. In a separate bowl, combine all of the wet ingredients. Make sure that the coconut oil is melted.

5. Mix the dry and wet ingredients and fold in the bacon crumbs gently. Do not over stir. Fold in well enough to be combined thoroughly. This is now your cookie mixture.

6. Form small balls using your hands and place them on the cookie sheet. Bake for about 8-10 minutes or until it becomes brown on top. Store in refrigerator or airtight container until ready to consume.

Nuts and Seeds Granola Bar

Ingredients

- 1 cup of walnuts (raw)
- 1 ½ cups of almonds (raw)
- 1 cup of pumpkin seeds (raw or sprouted)
- ½ cup of sesame and flax seed combo
- 1 cup of shredded coconut (unsweetened)
- 1 teaspoon of cinnamon
- 2 tablespoons of water
- 3 tablespoons of coconut oil
- 1 teaspoon of vanilla extract
- ½ teaspoon of cinnamon (ground)
- ½ teaspoon of kosher salt
- 1 egg (beaten lightly)

Directions

1. Preheat your oven to 300 degrees.
2. Line your baking tray using a parchment paper.

3. Place the walnuts, almonds and pumpkin seeds inside the blender or food processor. Pulse a few times until it becomes finely chopped. Makes sure not to grind them into a subtle texture.

4. On a large sized mixing bowl, whisk egg white with water until it becomes bubbly and a bit foamy. Add vanilla extract, salt, and cinnamon and whisk well.

5. Pour in the chopped nuts and seeds together with the shredded coconut. Mix well until everything is evenly coated.

6. Spread the mixture evenly on the lined baking pan. Bake for around 40 minutes or until it becomes crispy and golden brown. Stir it twice.

7. Remove from the oven and allow to cool for about 10 minutes. Using your spatula, scrape the granola and release the large clusters. Once cooled, store it in a resealable plastic or airtight glass jar.

8. Serve it on top of coconut yogurt with fruits, or you can add dried fruit.

Spicy Jicama Shoestring Fries

Ingredients:

- 1 piece of large Jicama (spiralized into noodles)
- 2 tablespoons of olive oil for drizzling
- Pinch of salt to taste
- 1 tablespoon of powdered onion
- 2 tablespoons of cayenne pepper
- 2 tablespoons of powdered chili

Directions

1. Preheat your oven to 405 degrees.
2. Place your Jicama noodles on a baking tray and cut them into small sized noodles making them look like shoestring fries.
3. Drizzle them with olive oil and lightly toss to evenly coat the noodles.
4. Season the Jicama noodles with salt, cayenne pepper, powdered onion and powdered chili. Again lightly toss them so that the spices and seasoning

will be evenly distributed. Make sure not to overcrowd the noodles to avoid sticking together.

5. Bake for 15 minutes then turn it over to bake them again for another 10 to minutes or until your preferred crispiness.

6. Store in an airtight container until 3 days.

Breakfast Porridge

Ingredients

- ½ cup of wild or red rice
- ½ cup of oats (choose the steel-cut ones)
- ¼ cup of faro or pearl barley
- ½ cup of wheat cereal or farina
- 1 piece of orange peel (cut to 2-inch slices)
- 1 part of cinnamon stick
- 1-2 tablespoons of brown sugar (choose from dark or light color)
- ¼ teaspoon of salt
- ¼ cup of dried fruit (pick your favorite fruits)
- 5 cups of water
- Chopped nuts, milk or maple syrup to serve (optional)

Directions

1. 12 hours before serving, you can prepare this dish in time for breakfast. Place rice, barley, farina, and oats inside the slow cooker. Mix in cinnamon stick, salt, sugar, 5 cups of water and orange peel. Add also the dried fruit of your choice.

2. Set the slow cooker for the porridge cycle, such that it will be cooked and prepared once you wake up in the morning. If you don't have a porridge cycle, you can cook for about an hour and warm them in the morning.

3. Serve with syrup or milk, top with nuts if you prefer.

Baked Chicken with Sweet Potato

Ingredients

- 6 cloves of diced garlic

- 2 tbsps of olive oil

- 1 large sweet potato, cut to an inch piece

- 2 cups of carrots, chopped to an inch piece

- 1 ½ cup of diced onions

- 1 lb of chicken breast, cut to an inch piece (raw)

- 1 lb of steamed broccoli

- 1 tsp of rosemary, dried

- ½ cup of parmesan

Directions

1. Preheat your oven to 375 degrees F.

2. Using a large baking tray, place garlic, olive oil, sweet potato, onion, carrots, chicken, plus rosemary. Season with a right amount of pepper and salt then

bake for around 30 to 40 minutes or until the chicken is cooked thoroughly and the veggies as well.

3. Add broccoli then parmesan. Place into individual containers.

Pear Noodles with Yogurt Parfait

Ingredients

- Greek yogurt (any flavor of your preference)

- 2 pieces of medium pears

- ¾ cup of diced fruits (mix of strawberries, bananas, and blueberries)

- 1 bowl of your favorite granola

Directions

1. Divide the mixed diced fruit into 3 separate mason jars. Top it with the yogurt then put 1/3 cup of granola in each pot.

2. Top the granola with the pear noodles. Refrigerate if you will not consume yet.

Breakfast Casserole

Ingredients

- A bag of 32 ounces of hash brown potatoes (frozen)
- 1 pound of bacon
- 1 piece of diced small onion
- 8 ounces of cheddar cheese sharp (shredded)
- ½ of diced bell pepper (red)
- ½ of diced bell pepper (green)
- 12 eggs
- 1 cup of milk

Directions

1. Slice bacon into small pieces and cook well. Drain excess fat.

2. Add half a bag of hash browns at the bottom of the crockpot then add half of the cooked bacon, half

onions, half of the red and green bell peppers and shredded cheese.

3. Place remaining half of hash browns on top. Followed by the remaining bacon, onions, cheese and the red and green bell peppers.

4. Meanwhile, crack 12 eggs in a bowl and whisk together with the milk. Pour this mixture into the crockpot and add pepper and salt.

5. Cook the mixture for 4 hours on low.

Easy Pea-sy Soup

Ingredients

- ½ cup of fresh parsley (chopped; plus add 8-10 parsley stems more)
- 4 sprigs of thyme
- 1 pound of green split peas (rinsed and picked over)
- 1 sizeable sized leek (use the light green and white part only; halved and sliced thinly)
- 2 stalks of chopped celery
- 2 pieces of carrots (chopped)
- Salt and pepper
- 1 smoked leg of turkey (around 1to 1 ½ pounds)
- ¼ cup of plain yogurt (non-fat)
- ½ cup of frozen peas (thawed)
- Crusty bread to serve (optional)

Directions

1. Tie thyme together with parsley stems using a kitchen string. Place it in the slow cooker. Add leek,

split peas, carrots, celery, a teaspoon of salt and half a teaspoon of pepper. Mix them to combine. Add turkey leg plus 7 cups of water then cover.

2. Cook on low for about 6-8 hours or until peas and turkey is tender. Once done, discard the twigs of herb. Discard bone and skin from the turkey then shred its meat.

3. Stir the soup vigorously to break peas and make soup smoother. You can add water if it is too thick for your preference.

4. Add about ¾ of the shredded turkey on the soup. Set aside a few types of meat for garnishing. Add chopped parsley and season with pepper and salt.

5. Ladle soup into serving bowls. Top with thawed green peas and meat. Serve with bread if you want. Serves 1.

Zucchini Salad with Spinach and Avocado Dressing

Ingredients

- ½ cup of edamame shelled

- 1 ½ cups of spiralized zucchini

- ½ cup of red bell pepper, chopped

- ½ cup of celery, sliced

- ½ cup of cherry tomatoes

- 2 tbsps of olives, optional

- ¼ cup of feta cheese, optional

For the dressing

- ½ of avocado

- ½ cup of spinach, packed

- 2 tbsps of Greek yogurt

- 2 tbsps of EVOO

- Juice of a lemon

- Pepper and salt for tasting

Directions

1. Mix all the dressing ingredients using the blender. Pour at the bottom of the mason jar.

2. Add the celery first then peppers, edamame, cheese, tomatoes, feta cheese and olives – following that order.

3. Lastly, put the zucchini noodles. Cover then refrigerate.

4. When ready to eat, shake the jar well and pour on a plate.

Curried Quinoa Salad

Ingredients

- 4 cups of water

- 2 cups of quinoa

- ½ cup of EVOO (extra virgin olive oil)

- 2 tbsps of curry powder

- ¼ cup of apple cider vinegar

- 2 small cloves of minced garlic

- 1 diced cucumber

- 1 lemon, juiced and zested

- 2 diced red bell peppers

- 2 diced green apples

- ¼ cup of thinly sliced basil leaves, sliced thinly

- Salt for tasting

Directions

1. Rinse quinoa then combines it with the curry powder, water, and salt in a large sized pot. Cover then bring to boil. Reduce the heat and continue to simmer for around 18 minutes. Remove from heat then let it stand for 5 more minutes.

2. Meanwhile, combine olive oil, salt, lemon zest and juice, vinegar and garlic. Whisk until combined well. Add the apple, peppers, and cucumber then add the warm quinoa and mix well. Let it sit for awhile until the liquid and flavors are well-absorbed.

3. Add basil then cover. Chill and transfer to plate or bowl when ready to the consumer. Makes around 6-8.

Chicken with Gravy Slow Cooker style

Ingredients

- 4-5 lbs of whole chicken
- 2 tablespoons ghee
- 2 medium-sized onions (chopped)
- 6 cloves peeled garlic
- 1 teaspoon of tomato paste
- ¼ cup of chicken stock
- ¼ cup of white wine
- Your favorite seasoning
- Kosher salt
- Fresh ground pepper

Directions

1. Prepare and chop all your vegetables.
2. Using a large-sized cast iron pan, melt ghee over medium to high heat. Sauté garlic and the onions. Add tomato paste. Cook for about 8-10 minutes and season the veggies with pepper and salt.

3. When all the veggies are lightly brown and soft, deglaze the pan with white wine and transfer everything in your slow cooker.

4. Meanwhile, season your chicken with pepper and salt and your favorite seasoning. Make sure to season them inside and out. Place the chicken, breast facing down inside the cooker. Cook on low heat for about 4-6 hours.

5. Once the cooking is done, take the chicken out and let it sit for about 20 minutes.

6. Take the excess fat on top of the vegetables inside the slow cooker. Using an immersion blender or hand blender, blend thoroughly until the mixture turned to a mouth-watering gravy. Adjust seasoning according to preference.

7. Slice or rip off your chicken using your hand's Place on a serving plate and put gravy on top of a small bowl.

Chia, Ginger and Grapefruit Pudding

Ingredients

For the pudding

- 6 to 7 tbsps of chia seeds

- 1 tsp of grated ginger

- ½ cup of canned coconut milk (full fat)

- 1 ½ cups of nondairy milk (unsweetened)

- 1 tsp of vanilla extract

- 1 to 3 tsp of maple syrup

For the topping

- ¼ cup of toasted coconut flakes, unsweetened

- 2 grapefruits, cut to segments

Directions

1. In a bowl, mix all the ingredients in the pudding. Cover then refrigerate for around 2 hours until it becomes thick. Shake or whisk occasionally. If the

dessert seemed to be thin after 2 hours, add more chia seeds, just 1 tablespoon letting it sit for another hour until it achieves a pudding-like texture.

2. Spoon in individual servings and top it with coconut and grapefruit. Makes about 2 servings.

Spiralized Zucchini with Corn and Tomatoes

Ingredients

- 4 medium size spiralized zucchini

- 2 ears of sweet corn (kernels removed from the cob)

- 1 pint of halved cherry tomatoes

- ½ cup of basil leaves

- ½ cup of Parmesan cheese shaved

- For the dressing

- ¼ cup of olive oil

- ¼ cup of grapeseed oil or any light oil

- ¼ cup of champagne vinegar

- ¼ tsp of sugar

- ½ tsp of kosher salt

- 1 clove of crushed garlic

Directions

1. Combine the corn, tomatoes, and zucchini in a bowl. Set aside.

2. Meanwhile, add all dressing ingredients in a jar and mix well. Add the zucchini mixture on top then place on the refrigerator. When ready to consume, shake well until thoroughly soaked.

3. Transfer to plate then top with cheese and basil. Serve.

Vegetarian Lasagna

Ingredients

- 1 26 oz jar of marinara sauce
- 1 14 ½ oz of canned diced tomatoes
- 1 8 oz pack of no-boil lasagna noodles
- 1 15 oz container of part-skimmed ricotta cheese
- 1 8 oz pack of mozzarella (shredded)
- 1 10 oz package of frozen spinach (thawed, chopped and squeezed to dry)
- 1 cup of veggie crumbles (frozen)

Directions

1. In a medium-sized bowl, combine tomatoes with its juice and marinara sauce.
2. Meanwhile, using a non-stick cooking spray, spray the bottom of the crockpot. Spoon a cup of tomato sauce mixture at the bottom.

3. Arrange ¼ of the noodles over the sauce. Overlap the noodles and make sure to break them to cover much of the sauce.

4. Spoon about ¾ cup of sauce on top of the noodles and top it with a half a cup of ricotta and half a cup of shredded mozzarella. Spread half of the spinach on top of the cheese.

5. Repeat doing the same process, twice beginning with the noodles. Once in the middle layer, replace the spinach using the frozen crumbles. Put remaining noodles and top it with the remaining sauce and cheese.

6. Cover and cook for about 2 ½ - 3 hours on low while 1 ½ - 2 hours on high or you can check to see if the noodles are already tender.

Egg and Veggie Cups

Ingredients

- 1 chopped red bell pepper

- 4 chopped green onions, use both white and green parts

- 8 eggs

- 1 tbsp of olive oil

- 1 chopped orange bell pepper

- Pepper and salt for tasting

Directions

1. Preheat your oven to about 350 degrees F.

2. Heat olive oil in large pan. Add the bell peppers, salt, and green onion. Sauté until veggies for around 5 to 7 minutes or until they are tender and soft. Remove and let cool.

3. Whisk together eggs and salt. Add sautéed veggies then mix well. Place mixture on greased muffin pans just enough to fill.

4. Bake for around 20 minutes or until it becomes puffy,

5. Remove from oven then let it cool. Serve, or it can be kept in the refrigerator in a sealed container for about 4 days. Makes about 12 egg and veggie cups.

Pecan, Cranberry and Orange Granola

Ingredients

- ¼ cup of orange juice

- 1 ½ cups of rice Krispies cereals

- 1 tsp of orange zest

- 1 ½ cups of old-fashioned oats

- ½ tbsp of oil

- 1 lightly beaten egg white

- 2 tbsps of maple syrup

- 2 tbsps of chopped pecans

- 3 tbsps of cranberries, dried

Directions

1. Preheat your oven to 350 degrees F then coat a square baking tray with non-stick spray.

2. Combine the oats with rice Krispies in a large sized bowl. Using another bowl, whisk the orange juice, oil,

egg white, maple syrup and orange zest. Pour in the cereal then stir with the spatula until it is coated evenly.

3. Spread on the baking tray and bake for around 40 to 45 minutes in the oven with 350 degrees F. Stir the mixture every 15 minutes or until it becomes crunchy and golden. Be sure to stir the granola to avoid getting burnt. Cool for around 5 minutes then adds in the pecans and cranberries. Store in a container.

Cashew Milk with Vanilla

Ingredients

- 3 cups of water

- 3 pitted Medjool dates

- 1 cup of raw cashews

- Pinch of salt, optional

- 1 tsp of vanilla extract

Directions

1. Blend in the cashews using a blender until it becomes powdery for around 30 seconds. Do not over blend or it will turn into cashew butter.

2. Add in pitted dates, water, and vanilla extract plus sea salt. Blend it again until it becomes smooth and well combined for around 30 seconds.

3. Store inside the refrigerator in a container that is sealed tightly. This will last for around 5 days.

Energizing Superfood Smoothie

Ingredients

- ½ of avocado

- 1 cup of coconut water

- ½ cup of kale

- ½ cup of tropical fruit (papaya, mango, pineapple or combination)

- ½ cup of spinach

- 1/3 cup of Greek yogurt

- 2 tablespoons of goji berries

- 2 tablespoons of cranberries (dried)

- 1 teaspoon of coconut oil

- 1 teaspoon of maca

- 1 tablespoon of coconut flakes

- 1 teaspoon of wheatgrass powder

- Sweeteners (this is optional; choose from honey, stevia or maple syrup)

Directions

Place all of the ingredients in your blender. Blend well until smooth. Transfer to a glass and enjoy!

Banana, Spinach, and Strawberry

Ingredients

- 2 cups of baby spinach

- 1 large sized banana

- A cup of water

- 4 large sliced strawberries

Directions

Place all of the ingredients in your blender. Blend well until smooth. Transfer to a glass and enjoy!

Kiwi and Banana Smoothie

Ingredients

- ½ cup of water

- 1 medium-sized banana (frozen or fresh)

- A cup of baby spinach

- 2 pieces of kiwi (cut to half and peeled)

- Sea salt

- ½ tablespoon of coconut oil

- A tablespoon of flax seeds or chia seeds

- A tablespoon of coconut flakes or shreds

- Sweeteners like maple syrup, honey or stevia (if desired)

Directions

Place all of the ingredients in your blender. Blend well until smooth. Transfer to a glass and enjoy!

Banana Superfood Smoothie

Ingredients

- 1 medium-sized banana (frozen or fresh)

- A cup of spinach

- 1 ½ cups of almond milk

- ½ cup of strawberries (frozen or fresh)

- 2 tablespoons of Greek yogurt

- ½ cup of mango chunks (frozen or fresh)

- A tablespoon of coconut oil

- A tablespoon of bee pollen

- A tablespoon of chia seed gel or chia seeds

- A cup of kale

- 1 tablespoon of gelatin (you can also use your protein powder)

- 1 tablespoon of hemp seeds

- Any other superfoods that you have (optional)

Directions

Place all of the ingredients in your blender. Blend well until smooth. Transfer to a glass and enjoy!

Orange and Carrot Smoothie

Ingredients

- 2 pieces of peeled clementines

- 4 pieces of shredded carrots (this should be about 2 cups)

- 2/3 cup of Greek yogurt (vanilla)

- A cup of romaine lettuce (chopped)

- ½ cup of ice cubes

Directions

Place all of the ingredients in your blender. Blend well until smooth. Transfer to a glass and enjoy!

Fruity Power Smoothie

Ingredients

- 2 cups of watermelon (cubed and seeded, rinds removed)

- 1 ½ cups of frozen strawberries (unsweetened)

- 1 ½ cup of small-sized cauliflower (florets only)

- 1 (6 oz) Greek yogurt (strawberry flavored)

- 2 tablespoons of strawberry preserves (if desired)

Directions

1. Using a small-sized saucepan cook the cauliflower for around 10 minutes or till it becomes very tender. Drain then rinse with cold water.

2. Place the cooked cauliflower, strawberries, yogurt, watermelon and strawberry preserves if you will use it. Cover then blend until smooth. Pour into a tall glass. Serve and enjoy!

CONCLUSION

You have finished reading this book. I hope you have learned so much and eventually make meal prepping a habit of your own. You see how beautiful meal prepping is? Take your time and be not afraid to start little by little. Remember that you don't have to prep it all. If you are just a beginner, this will be overwhelming for you. Just try to prepare meals that are good for only a day or two. Don't jump right away into preparing meals all for one week. Once you get comfortable with the process, everything will be easy breezy.

Another reminder is to follow recipes first especially if you are not familiar with some of the ingredients and procedures. This will help in giving you confidence as you go along your meal prep habit. Just focus on preparing the meals ahead of time. Make this book as your guide in your prepping habit. Enjoy and include your family members as well especially your children in making the preparations. This will help them learn the basics at an early age and teach them how to eat healthily.

Finally, give yourself some time to get used to this process.

Remember, nothing is learned overnight. There will be some mishaps and mistakes but over time you will learn from them. Do not get discouraged if that happens. Take note that meal prep is about making it easier for you and provide your family a healthy meal every day, not make it stressful for you. So just take it easy. I am confident that you will be able to push through and be successful on this journey.

Again, thank you and have a healthy and happy meal prep journey!

Final Words

Thank you again for purchasing this book!

I really hope this book is able to help you.

The next step is for you to **join our email newsletter** to receive updates on any upcoming new book releases or promotions. You can sign-up for free and as a bonus, you will also receive our "*7 Fitness Mistakes You Don't Know You're Making*" book! This bonus book breaks down many of the most common fitness mistakes and will demystify many of the complexities and science of getting into shape. Having all this fitness knowledge and science organized into an actionable step-by-step book will help you get started in the right direction in your fitness journey! To join our free email newsletter and grab your free book, please visit the link and signup: **www.hmwpublishing.com/gift**

Finally, if you enjoyed this book, then I would like to ask you for a favor, would you be kind enough to leave a review for this book? It would be greatly appreciated!

Thank you and good luck in your journey!

ABOUT THE CO-AUTHOR

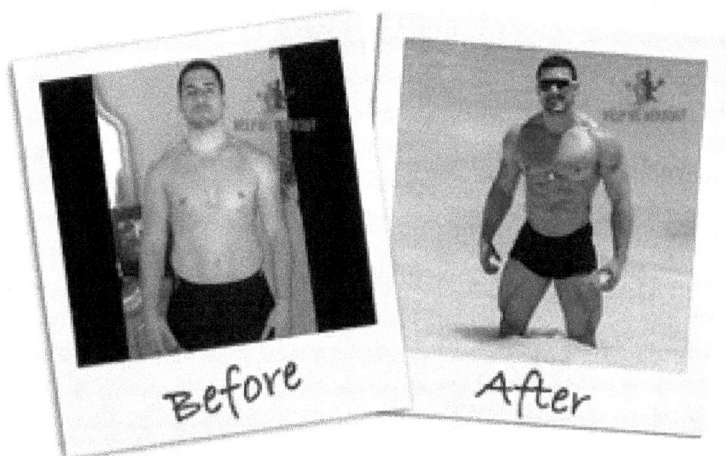

My name is George Kaplo; I'm a certified personal trainer from Montreal, Canada. I'll start off by saying I'm not the biggest guy you will ever meet and this has never really been my goal. In fact, I started working out to overcome my biggest insecurity when I was younger, which was my self-confidence. This was due to my height measuring only 5 foot 5 inches (168cm), it pushed me down to attempt anything I ever wanted to achieve in life. You may be going through some challenges right now, or you may simply want to get fit, and I can certainly relate.

For me personally, I was always kind of interested in the health & fitness world and wanted to gain some muscle due to the numerous bullying in my teenage years about my height and my overweight body. I figured I couldn't do anything about my height, but I sure can do something about how my body looked like. This was the beginning of my transformation journey. I had no idea where to start, but I just got started. I felt worried and afraid at times that other people would make fun of me for doing the exercises the wrong way. I always wished I had a friend that was next to me who was knowledgeable enough to help me get started and "show me the ropes."

After a lot of work, studying and countless trial and errors. Some people began to notice how I was getting more fit and how I was starting to form a keen interest in the topic. This led many friends and new faces to come to me and ask me for fitness advice. At first, it seemed odd when people asked me to help them get in shape. But what kept me going is when they started to see changes in their own body and told me it's the first time that they saw real results!

From there, more people kept coming to me, and it made me realize after so much reading and studying in this field that it did help me but it also allowed me to help others. I'm now a fully certified personal trainer and have trained numerous clients to date who have achieved amazing results.

Today, my brother Alex Kaplo (also a Certified Personal Trainer) and I own & operate this publishing venture, where we bring passionate and expert authors to write about health and fitness topics. We also run an online fitness website "HelpMeWorkout.com" and I would love to connect with by inviting you to visit the website on the following page and signing up to our e-mail newsletter (you will even get a free book). Last but not least, if you are in the position I was once in and you want some guidance, don't hesitate and ask... I'll be there to help you out!

Your friend and coach,

George Kaplo
Certified Personal Trainer

Get another book for Free

I want to thank you for purchasing this book and offer you another book (just as long and valuable as this book), "Health & Fitness Mistakes You Don't Know You're Making", completely free.

Visit the link below to signup and receive it:

www.hmwpublishing.com/gift

In this book, I will break down the most common health & fitness mistakes, you are probably committing right now, and I will reveal how you can easily get in the best shape of your life!

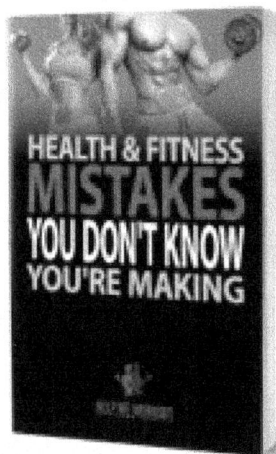

In addition to this valuable gift, you will also have an opportunity to get our new books for free, enter giveaways, and receive other valuable emails from me. Again, visit the link to sign up:

www.hmwpublishing.com/gift

HMW Publishing

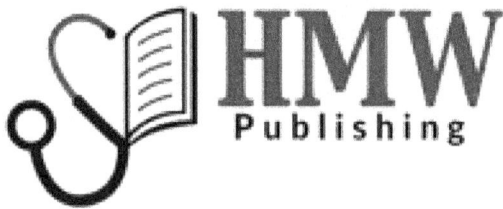

For more great books visit:

<u>HMWPublishing.com</u>

www.ingramcontent.com/pod-product-compliance
Lightning Source LLC
Chambersburg PA
CBHW050734030426
42336CB00012B/1568